Healing

7 Ways To Heal Your Body In 7 Days (With Only Your Mind)

RUTH LOGAN

CONTENTS

1   Introduction   6

2   Day 1 - Changing Limiting Beliefs   8

3   Day 2 - Listen to Your Body   11

4   Day 3 - Eliminate Stress   14

5   Day 4 - Manifestation   17

6   Day 5 – Visualization   20

7   Day 6 – Chakras   23

8   Day 7 – Reflection   25

9   Summary   30

    Other Books By Ruth Logan   31

HEALING

INTRODUCTION

Our minds are the most powerful tools in the universe, to help us heal quickly and with ease. Think about it for a moment, in this entire universe of stars, nebulae and galaxies, there is nothing as powerful as our mind, except for spirit. Modern medicine only worries about the mind when you have "lost it" and then treats it with chemicals, but that still doesn't cure the underlying problem.

Up until almost a hundred years ago, modern medicine consisted largely of the ingestion of certain chemicals or plants, without any clear understanding of what was wrong or how to fix it.

Modern medicine is a marvel, but the human brain, with all its capacity for thought and understanding is beyond marvelous and we would be doing ourselves a mighty disservice by not understanding how to use this tool to assist us in our own healing.

We need modern medicine to help us heal, but there is a point at which we can and must, take control and responsibility for our own health. That is by controlling our mind, one of the most important missing parts of the puzzle of health. We need to learn how to heal the headache and not just conceal it for a while with paracetamol, but understand where it comes from and our stressors and only then can we cure it. Our aim is to heal the cause not just the symptom.

If you need any proof of the strength of our mind in our healing, you only need to look at scientific evidence. Let's focus on the placebo experiment. Every test has two groups, one group gets given the actual medicine and the other group gets given a placebo, something like a sugar pill. What is found in many cases is that patients in a group that have been given the placebo also get better. This is called the placebo effect. Your mind is convinced that you are getting better from this "pill" and so you do.

There are even studies showing that the reverse is true. In the 1960's, tests by Rosenthal and Jacobson in the Oak School showed that children, conditioned to believe that they were superior in IQ, performed better than children who held no such belief, even though in fact they were lower in IQ. Our beliefs are incredibly strong and we need to use that knowledge to help our body to heal.

You have the ability to deal with illness in your mind, if it has been done by any human, with the same equipment as you (i.e. the mind), it can be done.

This book is a guide to helping your body heal with only the power of your mind. Your mind is the most powerful tool you have and you need to understand how it works and what influences it, in order to live as healthy and happy as you were meant to.

I've structured the book into 7 categories. You can focus on one topic a day or you can read the whole book and try several at a time. The intention in either scenario is for you to take action and start harnessing your mind's natural ability to heal itself.

You just need to believe in yourself, and this book will teach you how.

DAY 1 – CHANGING LIMITING BELIEFS

We all have subconscious limiting beliefs, hidden from our daily perspective which we don't realize limit us in ways we don't understand. For instance, perhaps you think that having your own business is bound to leave you broke eventually and it is much safer to work for someone. Hence, you keep working in a corporate environment which is not good for your mind and body and leaves you unfulfilled. You need to understand where this belief comes from, how you absorbed this. Perhaps your grandfather lost his business or you saw a family member constantly battle to make ends meet while working for themselves.

Once you are at the root of a belief, you can replace that belief with a positive one. Your grandfather might have lost everything, but that will make you more aware of the dangers of not budgeting and you will have the tools that he might not have had. You are able to look at what he had done, take the positive out of that and then use that to enable you in the process.

Often, a limiting belief is something that is rooted in the past, for instance something that you could not do because you were a child and incapable of handling the situation or were not trained to do it. However, now that you are older or better equipped to deal with it, you might find that you can do it easily once you understand that is only the fear that was holding you back.

You have taken a negative, examine the root and understand how to let that inform you in order to change it into a positive experience.

Eliminating negative beliefs is one of the best ways to clear your mind, and once you have dispelled them, you will realize that anything that can be done.

Meditation

Meditation has been proven to help with healing in so many ways. Studies have shown that people who regularly meditate have lower blood pressure, lower anxiety levels and panic attacks. The benefits are numerous and well published.

Although hard to explain, the ultimate aim of meditation is not to have an aim while meditating. Meditation is an absence of thought and having an aim is ultimately a thought, which would be beside the point of the exercise. When you meditate there is a space between thoughts, as it were. However, this is a long process which takes a lot of dedication and there are numerous ways of getting to that stage. Tools have been developed, over thousands of years, to assist us in reaching the point where there is a place between thoughts.

There have been many methods or techniques developed to assist with meditation. Using a word, to repeating a sound or even vigorous exercise before sitting down quietly and meditating.

Changing Limiting Beliefs

This technique will help guide your subconscious to identify your negative beliefs, eliminate them and replace them with positive new beliefs. This is of vital importance in the healing process, as we have to believe that healing can happen, but because of our conditioning over the years, we have to identify negative beliefs and eliminate them. Learn, unlearn and relearn.

It is important when you start to meditate to be dressed comfortably, sitting upright and warm. You need to be sure that you are relaxed, but not so much that you might fall asleep, which is why it is better to sit upright! If possible, try to mediate in nature where the sounds are soothing and there are no distractions, but if that is not possible, then mediate when there are no cars hooting in the streets outside or neighbors voices that can distract you.

If you are meditating at home, it is easier to meditate in a specific secluded area of your home, somewhere you will not be easily distracted with washing that needs to be done or a TV that is begging to be switched on.

Before you start meditating, bless your space, in whichever way you are comfortable with. Start by focusing on your breath. When you feel relaxed and ready, sit quietly and try to identify a fear or limiting belief. Once you have found it, follow its root back to where it might have originated, just like you would follow a ribbon lying on the floor to what might have caused it. If you get distracted, don't be frustrated, just go back to that thought and follow it through to its route again.

This might be slightly uncomfortable, because we all don't like looking our fears in the face, but stick with it, the discomfort is a learned behavior and when you learn to distance yourself from it, it will dissipate. Eventually you will find the thought or experience that started the limiting beliefs.

Once you have the belief in your mind, examine it gently. See where it might have come from. Then, as if the belief were a coin, flip it over and find the positive side. Nature loves balance and for every negative there will always be a positive. Find the positive, even if you have to dig deep. The easiest way to find the positive affirmation is to find actual proof of this. When you find the proof of a positive affirmation, your body will respond and then you are on your way to dispelling the negative thought completely.

DAY 2 – LISTEN TO YOUR BODY

Once you are able to eliminate negative beliefs, you will be able to start intuitively listening to your body without preconceptions that have been ingrained into your subconscious, through the conditioning absorbed either unconsciously or consciously, in your culture, family or friends.

Listening to your body is not just about taking note of pains and injury. Sometimes listening to your body is acknowledging that you get a reaction in your gut is a great way to control your inhibitions. When you start becoming more attentive to the messages that you receive from your body, your conscious brain starts to accept that it does not need an instant reaction.

When you trust that you can read the signals that are being sent to you through energy perception, the part of you that worries constantly: "Is this OK?" learns to quieten down, trusting that you will listen when there is a need to. It is no longer like the kid in the backseat, repeating the whole time: "Are we there? And now? And now?" making you want to drive into the closest bridge! It is a lot more relaxing way to live, because you are not constantly confused and primed for the unexpected.

Energy flows between people in different ways and understanding your body's energy response to people will help you to learn to trust it more in relation to your own health. Energy carries emotion with it and when you articulate the emotion, it is easier to identify the flow of energy.

Our bodies are composed from life energy that western doctors and researchers are still battling to understand. They can photograph it, so they now it's there, but they cannot explain it. Most doctors just file it under the "unknown" label, with idiopathic, and are content to just not know. However, some researchers and historians speculate that the halos that were painted around the ancient saints is an actual depiction of energy (the chakras), and the fact that this was done in both ancient Eastern and Western medicine is very intriguing. Even in South American drawings, some rulers were depicted with a golden disk around their heads.

The energy we use for healing is the energy that exists throughout the universe. Just as we are aware of magnetic fields but cannot see them, there is an energy that we are all subconsciously aware of, but cannot always see. Sometimes some people can see it clearly, but because it does not have a glowing neon sign with an arrow pointing to it, most people automatically assume they cannot see it. Sometimes, when we see a friend walking towards us, without understanding or even thinking about how we know, we can see they are off. We just unconsciously read their energy, without being able to articulate how.

Once you understand that our bodies are made of that energy, in Chinese medicine called chi, you need to visualize how this energy flows around your body and informs it. Inka shamans call these rivers of light "ceke". Eastern religions say that we have 7 chakras (the word chakras means "disk" in Sanskrit), or energy points based at 1) the bottom of the spine, 2) the pelvic area, 3) the solar plexus, 4) the heart, 5) the throat, 6) the pineal gland above our eyes and 7) the top of the scalp.

Often when you have an illness, there will be a blockage in that area, something like a swirling grey cloud, though people see it differently. This is where there is an energy blockage. Energy pools around this area, informs the body and we get ill.

When you are able to focus and start listening to your body, instead of drowning out the symptoms with noise and keep your focus from healing, you will be able to heal yourself with the healing light that is in all of us.

The Intuitive Healing Technique

Sit calmly, ready to meditate, bless your space and quietly focus your attention on your breathing. Once you are completely relaxed focus on the area where there is a problem, for instance if have lower back pain. Try to symbolically understand why you might have back problems ... perhaps you have too much weight on your shoulders? Perhaps you can't keep your back straight because of something you did? ... Recurring health problems often have symbolic cause and when you are able to see these causes and resolve them, you are then capable of permanently healing your body.

When you are healing a problem area in your body, you need to visualize this area, focus on it and bring your full attention to it. Once you can in your mind visualise the problem, the pooling of shadows, you need to send a white healing light to this chakra. This is where you heal your own body. Keep your focus on the area, let the light dissipate the shadows, back into the earth.

When you are finished, give thanks and relax.

DAY 3 – ELIMINATE STRESS

There is a reason that stress has been called "'the serial killer of the modern age". Stress causes up to 90% of health problems. It has been shown through studies that stress, even more than smoking or lack of exercise, causes heart disease. We take billions of dollars of pills to deal with its effects, we drink and are reckless to loosen its grip and still it finds and kills more people than can be calculated on the planet. The good news is that with a few shifts in our mindset, we can overcome any problems or issues relating to stress.

In order for you to heal from an illness, you need to understand what the stressors in your life are and how they are impactful to your health and well-being.

When we are in a stressful situation our bodies have a mechanism to deal with the stress. We have three organs (the hypothalamus, the pituitary gland and the adrenal glands, located at the top of the kidneys) that react by releasing two stress hormones, cortisol and adrenalin, directly into the bloodstream instead of sending the signals through the neo cortex, our logical brain.

Since the signals aren't sent straight into the logical brain, we can't stop to think when we are in imminent danger, we just react. These steroids allow the body to supply more energy, moving blood away from digestion and other non-vital functions by sending it to our major muscles in order to help us flee. These hormones are what allowed our forefathers to avoid danger, without having to think about it.

When an antelope is chased by a lion and escapes, his body reacts the same way. But he stands for a few moments, shaking all over and will then calmly continue grazing. His "flight or fight" button has been switched off, because if it was on the whole time he would not be calm enough to graze and his body instinctively knows the right thing to do.

Modern humans however, are stuck in chronic stressful situations where the "fight or flight" button is always on. We drive cursing in traffic and even though we are not in physical danger, our body is releasing the steroids because of threats it perceives, which are not real. Studies have shown that rats exposed to constant stress lose their ability to break out of repetitive behavior and become less creative and less cunning.

In the same way, humans who are constantly exposed to stress start to display repetitive behavior and are less capable of analytic thought. We start to feel like we are in a rut and develop symptoms of depression, unable to break out of the cycle. Because of the cortisol and adrenalin pumping through our bloodstream, it becomes impossible to change. We don't eat healthy, can't change bad behaviors and we chronically feel as if we are getting nowhere. This could lead to illness, which then causes more stress. The cycle continually repeats itself.

It is well known that in many instances stress can be reduced by exercise, healthy eating and drinking in strict moderation. However, when our bodies are not well, we have to look at other ways in which we can combat stress and lead us back to health. Even though stress might not be the cause of disease, being in a stressful situation does not assist healing at all and should be eliminated as much as possible.

Understanding the stressors in our lives

But first we have to understand the stressors in our daily lives. We tend to think that stress is caused by the high paced environment that is around us. By work and daily living. However, when you think about it for a few moments, there are some serious irregularities. Surgeons, who must have some of the most stressful jobs on the planet, do not necessarily have shorter life expectancies. If they did, hospitals would have them signing disclaimers too! Why would that be? A surgeon, who knows that someone's life depends on that person and is in theatre for 18 hours, should be one of the most stressed people on the planet.

This is another reason why we need to understand what our own stressors are. You need to be able to understand that although your job might be stressful, it is the fighting with your mother in law every week that is keeping your body in flight or fight. This is a process of elimination and careful thought. Do you get stressed driving to work, but sigh when you pull into the parking garage at work and then relax? Only to repeat the process again on the way to work? Understand your stressors, because only when you can consciously unpack them, can you start getting your body to switch off flight-or-fight.

Mindfulness Technique

The surest way to combat stress is by practicing mindfulness. Our egos like to keep us mired in yesterday's disappointments or tomorrow's worries.

The trick to being mindful is staying in the present moment. When you focus on what you are doing right now, it is hard to anticipate tomorrow's problems, or make judgments about yesterday's actions.

When you find yourself starting the spiral of worry, take 10 deep breaths … Breath in deeply, feeling the air rushing into your chest. You have to feel sure that the air has passed your lungs, through your torso and feel that your stomach is expanding. When you get to 10, exhale and refocus on your environment.

Another quick way to eliminate stress is finding 10 things to be grateful for, at that moment. Being grateful floods your bloodstream with endorphins, thereby negating the effects of stress and relaxing you instantly – works every time.

DAY 4 – MANIFESTATION

In order to manifest what we need, we have to align the entire body to our goal. This is not just a quick alignment that you forget after a moment what we are trying to do. Manifestation literally means the action or fact of showing something.

When you manifest something, you are focusing your entire intention on that subject. Your whole body and mind is dedicated to achieving a goal and trusting that it will become so with every fiber of your being.

If you think about an acorn, it does not have any other aim than to manifest as an oak tree – there just are no other options available to it. It's not thinking: "maybe a fig tree, or maybe fir … "It is going to become a mighty oak! Try to imagine how that must feel, the sureness of knowing what you are destined to be.

Understanding manifestations is knowing that we all have the power to manifest exactly that which we desire. That energy is in all of us. It is the cosmic energy that created the universe and as we are a part of the universe, that cosmic energy is in us as well. However, we can also unconsciously manifest - we can also pull that towards us which we do not desire. The law of attraction works both ways. So it is extremely important to consciously manifest our desires and avoid those phrases and habits that manifest those things that we do not want.

Try this experiment … **Don't** think of an elephant in ballet shoes … Do you see how that worked? It is not possible to <u>not</u> think of something negative. You have to retrain your brain to think differently. When you say something like "I will no longer be ill", the word ill (the negative) is the one the universe focusses on. Like attracts like. It is vitally important, when you are manifesting, to understand that you have to say 'I am happy, healthy and balanced" – focus on the positive, that is what the law of attraction will bring towards you, positive attracting positive.

You can also do verbal affirmations, many people do this as well and it is very helpful. However, unlike Captain Kirk, saying "Make it so!" does make a spaceship fly. Affirmations are only a tool to help with the manifestation. There are no shortcuts to knowing something, you either know or you hope. You have to know, from the middle of your solar plexus, that this is what you are meant to do.

Theta Night Sound Technique

From time immemorial, sound has played a huge part in the human experience. Ancient cultures used sound to elevate themselves into a religious trance. Even today, the quickest way we know how to calm ourselves is with the use of sound. You only need to see the effect of Beethoven on a baby to know that the baby is calm and attentive, and students have known for decades that listening to Mozart will help them study.

Like light, sound is made up of frequencies, and as such vibrates with the rhythm of the universe. One way of using these frequencies is to use theta waves to "tune in" to the universe, helping us to align with all energy, and enabling the manifestation process. The ancient Tibetans used the sound of prayer bowls to mediate and achieve a deeper state of relaxation. Kalahari bushmen would beat drums wildly and dance their way into the scared.

We all have heard of alpha and delta brainwaves: Alpha waves are when we are restful or dreaming in a REM cycle; Beta waves when we are concentrating or fearful. However there are also Delta waves when we are in dreamless sleep or unconscious; Gamma waves when we are solving intricate problems. Most importantly for us, there are also Theta waves, which is what we are in when we are mediating.

Theta waves can be listened to when we want to help us enter a deep state of consciousness, when we are meditating or manifesting. They are easy to download of the internet. Listen to them while you are either in a restful state or while meditating or manifesting a healthy, happy future.

DAY 5 – VISUALIZATION

A very important part of healing is the ability to visualize a different outcome. This has been used by ancient civilizations for centuries. Visualizing is not wishful thinking. When you wish for something, you take no personal responsibility for the outcome. But if you visualize, your intention has been established and when you visualize, you are taking responsibility for the process that allows your body to heal itself and be in a better state.

Visualizing is the holding of an image in your mind, informing your mind of the feeling and sensations and thus implanting the picture into your mind and body. Remember how our body deals with imagined stress, the way we deal with a stressful situation even though it is not really there? This is where we use the opposite of that process.

When we experience or imagine something good happening to us, our body releases endorphins, the feel good hormone which allows healing to occur faster and make us more relaxed. Because our mind does not differentiate between an actual event and an event that hasn't happened, but is only being imagined, our body reacts the same way to both events and this is why visualization works for us when we are trying to heal.

Visualizing is conscious dreaming, intentional. They are both extremely important. When you are visualizing you are consciously and intentionally giving your mind permission to play. You are painting pictures in your mind's eye with vivid colors and bold strokes, creating a world you can play in.

Day dreaming is not visualizing. When you day dream, your mind is not "switched on", there is no intent. So sitting day dreaming during a math class does not constitute visualization! Anything that is done unconsciously is of no real benefit, there is no alignment with the universe. When you are conscious about what you are doing, then the sparks start to fly!

Being mindful

However, you need to be aware. There is another kind of visualization. This is could be called unconscious visualization and when you have been ill for a while, this is where you unconscious thoughts usually go. Some people even call it a form of black magic, how we curse ourselves with our negative thoughts. These cycles continue in an endless, a repetitive chime about how bad things are, like the rats running through a maze, unable to break repetitive patterns.

When we imagine the worst outcome for a test or we imagine our spouse leaving us or an earthquake, again, our body does not know the difference between an actual event and an imagined event. Our body releases stress hormones and we feel anxious and while those hormones are floating around in our body, healing cannot happen. No matter how much you visualize healing for that concentrated period of time, you cancel that effect out during the course of the day when you, out of habit, imagine the worst of the situation.

It is very, very important to mind your thoughts, especially when you are tired or ill. But it can be done, it can be done because you are aware and you have control over those thoughts, especially the small ones.

When you catch yourself having a negative thought, cancel it out, do whatever helps you to replace it with a positive. You might put an elastic band around your wrist which you snap against your wrist when you have a negative thought, and then smile. You might repeat a phrase that you connect with, something positive and short that gives you instant hope. Try, find what works for you, you will stop eventually.

Cellular Influence Technique

When you are consciously visualizing, try to be in the same environment as you would be when you are meditating. Be comfortable and at ease. Visualizing is a lot more fun than meditating. Meditating is hard, takes a lot of practice to one day reach time when you become timeless, but extremely necessary to stop the negative thought cycle.

Imagine that you are happy healthy and loving life. Feel the sensation of health pulsing in your veins, muscles and skin. If your leg is hurt, imagine standing on a grassy field, running and feeling the grass underneath your feet. Put in as much detail as you can. Are you in a field, a park? Are there clouds outside floating past? Can you feel the grass tickling your hands when you do a handstand? Are there small flowers in the grass?

Include all images and sensations that can help you connect you to your visualization. This is what could be called conscious dreaming. The same way you wake up laughing from a dream, this is where your mind needs to be to be happy and release those endorphins! When your cells receive the endorphins, they do not know that they are not in a park, they know that they are healing. This is why it is so important to be fully immersed in it.

DAY 6 – CHAKRAS

Modern mystics and ancient sages have always understood that nothing in the universe exists in isolation. Just like we are atoms that exist in cells, cells that exist in organs, organs that exist in living beings, living beings that exist on earth, an earth which again exists in the universe, everything is linked in ways which we currently barely understand and cannot explain. A massive set of Russian dolls nestled into each other.

As we previously saw with energy healing, healing the entire body is a process of understanding how the affected chakra might influence our illness and how the symbolic meaning of illness can perhaps illuminate the cause of an illness. Energy healings as discussed in the previous chapter is looking at a specific area and sending the healing white light to that part to heal it.

What we are doing in this chapter is looking at the entire body, each chakra, for patterns that might be emerging in specific areas Perhaps you somehow always have problems with your feet, from a broken toe to a twisted ankle. There might be a link there, perhaps you are scared to stand on your two feet, or feeling insecure and not grounded? Look for the patterns, because that is what is going to inform you into the long term. This is what we are ultimately tracking, not just healing a symptom, but understanding a pattern in order to heal it.

By not just looking at the illness, but also understanding that there might be a corresponding problem within our chakra is one of the most important lessons that we have to learn. Medical intuitives such as Caroline Myss and Mona Lisa Schultz have both written very eloquently about the link between illness and an energy imbalance in the corresponding chakra. In fact, often it is by reading the chakras that they have picked up an unknown problem in the body.

For us to understand how this works, we need to pay more attention to the symbolic language that we use in our everyday speech. Our ancestors intuitively knew that they had a bad "gut" feeling, long before researchers investigating how moods, thoughts and emotions affect us, found neuropeptides in our bloodstream, affecting our bodies and emotions. The same chemicals that are in our brain are also in our bodies. These neuropeptides are found in our gut, hence a gut feeling.

Mind-Body Technique

When you are at ease and in a restful state of mind, start by imagining your chakras, one by one. You just need to imagine where your chakras are, and then feel how they vibrate. It sounds harder than it is, you have learnt how to focus and disregard negative emotions, and you are now just trying to find the energetic patterns which lead to illness. Instead of focusing on one area, what you are doing now is investigating the entire organism.

Let say you get an uncomfortable feeling when you look at the heart chakra. It makes sense, you have high blood pressure. You then get an uncomfortable feeling at your throat chakra as well. When you focus your thoughts, you remember that you often get laryngitis. Could the laryngitis be linked to the heart problem? And eventually, perhaps you could see that the anger against your mother in law makes you lose your voice because you don't want to fight. The correlation has been established, and now you know you are fixing the disease in its entirety, not just the symptoms. Healing can start fully.

Once you have received that message, thank your body for informing you what is toxic for you and let it go, the lesson has been learnt.

DAY 7 – REFLECTION

Once you have looked at your body and your illness as a symbiotic relationship, where your body / mind and illness feed off each other, you can understand how to avoid illness and how to reduce stress and increase every day well-being. This is of crucial importance, but there remains a bit of a hurdle before you will be able to be completely healed.

When you realize that your illness has become something that has informed you of a life lesson, you will reach the point where you can thank your body for that lesson, for helping you to discover the gift of life.

The ancient shamans would carry a bag of healing totems with them. These totems were a symbol of what illnesses and difficulties they knew they had overcome. They had learnt and been informed by their illnesses and troubles. As it has ben said: Courage is not the absence of fear, it is the overcoming of it. Once you have learnt that you can conquer a fear, you become more courageous because of it.

Life is never just a negative and when you are able to see the positive hidden in the folds of a negative, you are fully able to let the negative go, retain only the victory of the positive as a lesson learnt that you need not go over again.

Reflection Session

When you are at ease, sit quietly and observe your body, through your mind's eye. See your heart pumping rich blood through your veins, see the rise of your chest when you take a breath, feel the strength in your muscles. Thank your body for the lessons it has brought you, for the duties it performs every day in your honour, even without you knowing it.

Let's Reflect on Day 1:

You should've changed some of your limiting beliefs that stop you from achieving your goals and becoming fulfilled. If you are still facing issues, try writing your thoughts down and get to the root of the issue by asking yourself why you feel a certain way about it. Once you understand why, you'll find it easier to come to terms with it and bin it from your subconscious mind. Once, this stage is complete, begin meditating again.

Let's Reflect on Day 2:

Listening intuitively to your body is very often overlooked and dismissed. However, it is a vital part of the healing process. While meditating try to focus your energy onto the problem area. If this method isn't working, then visualize yourself healing before you use the meditation technique to get your mind prepared and energized.

Let's Reflect on Day 3:

Stress is the ultimate health inhibitor. It causes up to 90& of all health problems and it's no wonder why. We're under huge amounts of stress from our hectic daily lives. That is why it's so important to control and eliminate as much of it as you can. The mindfulness technique helps you focus on the present and not on the future which causes us the most amount of worry. Once you master this being in the present, it'll help take you out of the situation to calm yourself and elevate the pressure. If you're having trouble with this technique, don't give up! It'll take time and a lot of mental strength. So, practice every time you enter a stressful mental situation.

Let's Reflect on Day 4:

You have the ability to manifest any result that you desire. You just need to align your entire body with the goal. The sound technique will make it easier for you to achieve this. You should by now, have your body moving at the same frequency as your goal. If you're having issues with attaining your desired outcome, then try listening to a different frequency of sound for your body to flow with. Once, you get to the ideal frequency on a level in which your body can connect with, you'll be on your way to achieving any positive result in no time.

Let's Reflect on Day 5:

Visualization is a really beneficial skill to acquire. You need to envision a positive result before you can achieve it. Affirm your mind with the attributes of your desired outcome. Your mind will be in a positive state, which in turn affects your body.

We usually tend to envision negative outcomes as a way to protect ourselves, but that is a bad trait that we carry and need to unlearn it to allow only positive thought into our subconscious (the one we can't control).

Get into a positive and comfortable environment before you start using the technique. If you're having trouble with visualizing only positive things then try lighting your favorite candle in that room to appeal to your senses. It's been proven to help. Visualization is a skill that is acquired and so may not come quickly and easily to you. But, that's ok as long as you practice often.

Let's Reflect on Day 6:

There are 7 chakras: each to keep our bodies in balance.

Heart Chakra – Is associated with our faculty to love. It is centred in the middle of the chest, above heart. Bearing emotional issues with inner peace, joy and love.

Throat Chakra – Is associated with our faculty to communicate. Situated in the throat. Bearing emotional issues with self-expression, communicating your feeling or talking in general.

Third Eye Chakra – Correlates with our ability to focus on and see the larger picture. This chakra is situated between the eyebrows. Bearing emotional issues with the ability to think for oneself and make decisive choices, Intuition.

Crown Chakra – Is the highest chakra as it has the ability to connect to your highest spiritual power. The chakra is situated at the top of the head, where the crown is. Bearing emotional issues, such as; inner and outer beauty, calmness and our connection to our own spirituality.

Root Chakra – Is the chakra that represents us being grounded and stable. It is situated at the bottom of the spine where the tailbone is. Bearing emotional and survival issues, such as; money for supplies and financial independence.

Sacral Chakra – Is our ability to connect with people and create new experiences. It is situated on the lower abdomen. For bearing emotional issues, such as; well-being, being abundant, well-being.

Solar Plexus Chakra – Our ability to be in control of our lives confident and in-control of our lives. Location: Upper abdomen in the stomach area. Emotional issues: Self-worth, self-confidence, self-esteem.

Each represents a targeted problem that is associated with a healing chakra method. Take perspective of the chakra that's mirroring your issue, that way you can focus on healing that specific problem area solely to cure it entirely.

Look at what has worked for you when exploring these chakras and if in some areas you're not improving or getting your desired result then put all of your healing energy into one chakra, a day at a time until you see a positive result. It may also be helpful to listen to calming music with no influences of speech.

Your thoughts affect you on a physical level, so it's important that you write them off, otherwise your desired outcome may be at stake.

Open up your chakras to unleash endless possibility, wellness and regained health. You will only have one body in this lifetime, treat it always with gratefulness and respect.

SUMMARY

This book has been written with the aim of helping you heal your body with your mind in 7 days. I hope it acts as the initial step towards the excellent health you deserve. When you understand how to break free from thoughts that only limit you, that do nothing but stop you from moving forward, you will start reclaiming your health back.

The art of meditating and visualization are life skills, every bit is as important as knowing how to count, perhaps more so, because they connect us to a place that is timeless and a future that is limitless. Please be patient. These techniques will take time to learn and develop. Once you start to feel the benefits of these techniques and practices, I encourage you to further your reading in each area. You can start with the one that has benefitted you most during these 7 days.

You can do anything in this life that you want to, but the old adage remains true always: You have to put your mind to it.

OTHER BOOKS BY RUTH LOGAN

Limiting Beliefs - 7 Ways To Stop Limiting Beliefs In 7 Days

Gratitude - 7 Steps To Feeling More Grateful In 7 Days

www.ingramcontent.com/pod-product-compliance
Lightning Source LLC
Chambersburg PA
CBHW070940290526
45795CB00003B/1087